Chiropractic Concepts In Healing

Frank Zolli, D.C.

Printed in the United States of America

ISBNO-938470-01-9

Published by
NEW YORK CHIROPRACTIC COLLEGE
OLD BROOKVILLE, NEW YORK 11545

DEDICATION

I have found, having spent some twenty years in school, that too much emphasis is put on education, and not enough is put on learning. The best learning occurs when a student is able to observe a master at work and that student absorbs every lesson the teacher can give.

In my life, I have been fortunate to have two masterful teachers. For their years of devotion and toil, I dedicate this book, with love and respect, to my mother and father.

The author wishes to acknowledge those individuals whose critical, creative and technical skills contributed to the production of this book.

Salvatore Agro, Ph.D.
Mrs. Alice Agro
Mrs. Arlene Federico
Ms. Carla Lorenz
Ms. Angela Zolli
Alexander Zolli, M.D.

Special thanks to Adelia Russo, for everything.

ABOUT THE AUTHOR

Frank Zolli, D.C. was born and raised in Jersey City, New Jersey. He graduated from St. Peter's College with a B.S. in Psychology before entering Columbia Institute of Chiropractic. He is presently a member of the faculty of the New York Chiropractic College. Dr. Zolli also maintains private practices in Jersey City and Oceanside, New York.

HISTORY IS BUT THE STORY OF THE ACHIEVEMENTS OF PEOPLE WHO HAD CREATIVE IMAGINATION.

INTRODUCTION

The body is a complex, interrelated, interdependent unit. The neuroendocrine system is primarily responsible for this miraculous interplay. We owe a great tribute to the early pioneers of the chiropractic profession who paid the personal price for developing, adhering to, disseminating and propagating the revolutionary concept of natural healing called chiropractic. In spite of social denigration, including incarceration, these early doctors of chiropractic persisted and were rewarded by sick people getting well even when all else had failed.

There is a growing tendency by recent graduates to emphasize the diagnostic, laboratory and other modern technologies while frequently forgetting the basic clinical concepts of chiropractic. This is often at the expense of the patient's health and finances.

The author, Dr. Frank Zolli, has perceived this trend and hopes to get the students and all others in our profession back to basics with an appreciation of the natural principles upon which chiropractic is based. Once achieved, this knowledge of the inherent recuperative ability of the body, coupled with logical thinking, allows the profession to devote itself to the study of the "whole man" and not to this system or that organ, thereby neglecting the neurophysiological processes which help the sick get well by chiropractic principles and practice.

The failure of drugs, surgery, and other invasive procedures to help the patient offers chiropractors the opportunity to prove themselves worthy of partnership in the health care delivery system of tomorrow.

Dr. Zolli is to be complimented for his searching of our "roots" and demonstrating how modern and contemporary these principles truly are.

A.E. Cianciulli, D.C.

PREFACE

A Touch of Philosophy

In our relationships with people, we find that they divide themselves into two basic classes: Those who are superstitious, theoretical, believing in the mysterious. While they do not define it, their daily lives portray that of the visionary, flighty and hysterical. Then there are those individuals who believe in things that are practical, who reason everything carefully - the matter of fact person who wants to know before taking any action.

I am personally acquainted with people who are very practical when dealing with therapeutical questions, but extremely superstitious in theological matters. There are certain problems we are all required to face which are common to mankind. One may be a good financier and make money rapidly, yet lack judgement in gambling. Which category to place these men in is speculative.

Each type thinks and acts those things which he does or does not deduce. The individual who is superstitious or whose mind tends in that direction will act so in his daily life. The very first thing in the morning he will say, "There is a spider in the corner. I will experience misfortunes today." Everything implies good or bad luck. The other type of individual will reason things out. He may step on a thousand spiders --- that act could not make clouds shed water. The fault of the existence of these types lies not only with ourselves but with education of the past. We were not taught to reason. Superstitions are easier than fact --- therefore, today we have an abundance of non-essential theories prevailing where there should be truth if we were to reason.

One word comes to my mind particularly at this time --- CHANCE - - Chance means hazard, risk, danger, uncertainty, insecurity, unreliable, perhaps, etc. It spells thought that may not be justifiable for our actions. Do you realize how few people think and how many act the life of chance?

There are people who would not start a job on Friday; others who would not sleep in berth thirteen. I know one man who carries a rabbit's foot; another a horse chestnut. Why? Good luck superstition. All of these acts are mysterious because there is no reason.

People are doing things by chance because of customs, style -- oftentimes they themselves consider it to be proper. I mention these instances to indicate that the external duties of personal life are for the most part governed by ideas of superstition and mystery. It is only one step from the thought and idea of chancing one's financial life. As a result, we have games of chance, roulette, cards, dice, horse racing and slot machines. There is another chance that people take in relationship to their health. How many people believe that gold earrings will improve sight -- that copper wire around the wrist will prevent rheumatism -- that only medicine will cure -- that whiskey is good for everything -- that the moon affects the mind? These and many more myths make up the fragmentary creeds of health that we have inherited.

There was a time when all stores and retail outlets practiced "Caveat Emptor". 'Let the buyer beware'-- that sign should be placed in every professional person's office. Beware of what you buy and investigate before you take anything into your body. If each individual would do just that it would drive one class out of business and simplify education for the other.

Principle means a great deal to some people and very little to others. Principle, law, reason, logic, intent, truth, confidence and reliability are synonymous. They seldom reason what they are thinking. They are on a time track -- seldom do they question right or wrong. People have a tendency to condemn that which they are ignorant of and endorse their prejudices.

Every thought and action should be self-analyzed and self-tested - mentally and physically. We should prove correct every action before we follow; it should contain the elements of fact and truth; it should be logical before we accept it. How many people can say that they are conscientiously performing in their daily lives in that manner? If you believe that you are, follow this suggestion tomorrow: Question everything before you do it and determine if you would have followed the same path if you automatically acted. I feel certain that you will experience a modification of your daily activities and participation.

Under the heading of principle we discuss generalities of life and how they should be guided by reason. It is a blend -- gradation from generalities of life to that which we now draw close to the financial consideration of principle. We all work more or less for something; perhaps for riches. How are you doing this? Will you succeed? If you are working for money there is only one way that you could be successful. Make your foundation the attaining of some other and based upon principled delivery and as a result the following thoughts will grow.

You grow rich when you earn what you give. You receive in ratio as you give. You accumulate as you labor. You will be rich in storage, in ratio to that which you dispense to your fellow man. You will know in thought that which you give in action. You take what others give, by what you give them. You cannot keep the dollar you have not earned. Reciprocity makes for wealth.

The storehouse of success resides within you in what you give to the world. As we work diligently to earn, as a matter of principle, so must we discipline ourselves to learn, as a matter of principle. We never accumulate knowledge unless we conscientiously apply ourselves. As we analyze how to gain wealth so must we analyze how to get well. Principle is that condition which forges the reason, blazes the path, constructs the vehicle, and delivers the product.

Low back trouble, torticollis, and headaches are effects. Principle says there is a cause. Life and death are contrasts on opposite extremes. Principle states there are multiple variations between life and death. Principle states we are born complete and should live altogether and die of old age the same way. Principle states we are a unit sufficient within ourselves, except for the air we breathe, water we drink and food we eat. Life comes at birth; stays with us until death. Life and disease are comparative in degree. To increase one is to decrease the other. Principle says life is within oneself - not in anything else. Principle says if there is an effect there is a cause. Locate the cause and correct it. If the cause is corrected there is life -- the correction of cause removes the effect. The principle is universal.

When a Chiropractor deals with that idea he is obliterating any chance. History has many roles, but law is eternal. Law in man is innate intelligence. You are not working with innate but permitting it to personify natural created objects -- your desire is that innate manifest itself in the composite compilation. In doing this you trifle with no game of chance ---- THIS IS PRINCIPLE.

Chiropractically speaking, getting well is a legitimate reaction with favorable odds. Every adjustment given increases the profits of both the patient and the Doctor of Chiropractic - for no matter how much the Chiropractor gives, the patient stands to receive more. The Chiropractor has removed no organ or tissue; disturbed no structure. He has permitted to be restored that which the patient needed -- intelligent selection of health residual in the body. This is not totally true of other therapeutics or any game of chance.

From the ruins of failures, arises the tower of success. Brick is made of dust which might have once been brick. The Chiropractor's success, is in part, due to the failure of other therapies.

If other therapies were not procedures of chance, Chiropractic would not have survived. Some are of the opinion that Chiropractic is valid for only one disease in one part of man -- the low back. It is a principle with which we work. It is broad enough for all the world and everything in it. The only difference between any disease is degree of effect -- which is dependent upon the degree of subluxations and degree of nerve involvement and the limitation of matter.

Why allow degree to change all which should be principle in your mind, into chance in practice? The universal principle is found everywhere, in all things, at all times.

Innate is universal to all objects of composite purpose. Why not use good common sense with yourself. The Chiropractor knows each person is subject to law common to all. Law, being within the person, adapts itself to the peculiar manners of living, etc. - ad infinitum of each individual. That law works within the patient, not the Chiropractor or anything else. This takes place within the patient, from the common source which flows through him as it does each of us. Knowing this, it is easy to find the spine, locate the subluxation, and adjust according to an infinite rule which could not vary, regardless of how much one would like it to.

We could not find a subluxation that does not exist. We could not produce a subluxation if we desired. We could not pervert currents into wrong acts if we wished. All we do is correct that which is out of plumb. Once this is done, our endeavors are at an end. From that time on, law does what is required to improve health.

Many look at Chiropractic as though it were a game of chance, good for some conditions and not for others; all right as far as it goes, but it does not go far enough. But on closer inspection, it does not resolve into that. It is applicable to all things, under all conditions.

Resolve your mind's efforts into the study of Principle. Study Principle and you will not ask chance questions. Chance says "maybe" but principle says "two times two is four" - not sometimes but always.

Is Chiropractic a game of chance or a principle and practice? I respond by asking, "Will oil mix with water?" "Will chance and principle cohabit?" "Will they mix in theory and practice?" No - neither will chance -- study and theory -- and practice, mix with the principle of study and practice.

It is with a sense of humility and gratitude that I express my appreciation to Dr. Frank Zolli for inviting me to present this Touch of Philosophy in his book -- CHIROPRACTIC CONCEPTS IN HEALING. He is a man who truly has the big idea.

Ernest G. Napolitano, D.C.

Table of Contents

AMONG ALL PEOPLES

AND IN EVERY AGE,

NOTHING HAS BEEN SO

PERSISTENTLY SOUGHT

AS BODILY HEALTH.

PROLOGUE

Chiropractic students today are unlike their predecessors. They have entered a profession that has established itself in the health care delivery system. They are faced with the prospect of financial reward and societal respect if they ethically practice their chiropractic principles. No longer is the profession shunned by the public. No student today will have to fear being jailed for practicing chiropractic. That privilege has become a matter of chiropractic history, a medal of honor for pioneer chiropractors who put their lives and their livelihood on the line to preserve the principles and practice of chiropractic. Those men and women, who did not possess the in-depth textbook knowledge of subjects that today's students are expected to maintain, practiced chiropractic before it was fashionable. Those doctors of chiropractic were able to help chiropractic grow by applying chiropractic principles to those patients entrusted to their care and getting results.

The students of today have reaped the rewards of chiropractic pioneers. Today, however, they are faced with new challenges that stalk the profession. Chiropractic has achieved success in gaining public, professional, and government recognition, due to dedicated individuals who, in true chiropractic tradition, sacrificed their time, effort, and part of their lives, so chiropractic could assume its rightful place in the healing arts. Because of their success, there is a tendency for the new breed of chiropractors to be somewhat complacent. The battle to establish chiropractic as a legitimate and singificant force in the health care delivery system has been won. Now effort must be expended to maintain the victory that has taken a long time to achieve.

Chiropractic will be able to maintain its rightful place as an integral part of the healing arts by continuing its productive record of success in the treatment of patients. The treatment of these patients will be the direct result of how chiropractic students are taught to be chiropractors. The future of chiropractic has been entrusted to chiropractic educators. Their orientation in patient management will influence the direction chiropractic moves in the future.

There is more and more visible evidence that the allopathic profession has been inadequate in satisfying the needs of the public. This can be attributed to the limited causality concept by which they practice. The allopath has centered the treatment of the sick on a strictly scientific approach. As there are many reasons for disease to occur, there are many factors that influence a disease state. To approach a complex dilemma from a single point of view, and attempt to correct this problem with singular orientation, is to limit the effectiveness of treatment.

In addition to other differences between the chiropractic and allopathic professions, the orientation with which doctors approach patients is the most deep seated. Chiropractors possess the same basic science background as allopaths, but the orientation is different. Whereas allopaths flounder in a sea of haphazard scientific miracles, chiropractors are guided by the principles and philosophy with which the profession has grown.

The best way to achieve a successful record of treating patients is by the proper clinical application of chiropractic principles. The only way to insure this proper clinical application is by having an in-depth, intimate knowledge of these principles.

At one time, when the educational process was not as sophisticated as it is today, chiropractic students entered school because they or members of their families were helped by chiropractic. They had a first-hand knowledge that chiropractic worked. They may not have understood the significance of an adjustment or how it works, but they could not deny the results.

Nowadays, many students enter school primarily with the intention of seeking fame and fortune by becoming a doctor. Their knowledge of chiropractic is based on reading some literature that briefly describes what chiropractic is. They have no idea what the science, art, and philosophy of chiropractic is all about. They cannot personally relate to the stories and accounts of seemingly miraculous chiropractic achievements. Today's students are the products of many years of exposure to medical propaganda. From their earliest days of watching television and looking through magazines they have "learned" of the miracle effect of drugs. These students, because they lack a personal affiliation with chiropractic, are skeptical of its value. They hear stories of how effective chiropractic has been in treating difficult cases and smile condescendingly, with some hidden knowledge that, if the patient had been correctly treated by a medical doctor, chiropractic intervention would not have been necessary. These are the same students who in a matter of four short years enter society as chiropractors. In that time, a transformation from skeptic to believer must be made. Societal influence being what it is, this transformation is not an easy accomplishment.

Old fashioned chiropractors were deep-rooted in the principles of chiropractic. They were taught to be chiropractors when education was not standardized. Formal training could last from six to eighteen months. The accumulated knowledge of anatomy and physiology was not as extensive as present information. The most consistent part of chiropractic training at that time was the study of chiropractic principles. Because the basic science information was limited, diagnostic skills were limited. Therefore, the clinical rationale for treatment was a combination of the available anatomical and physiological data with a thorough knowledge of chiropractic pinciples.

Today, in a highly sophisticated, technical world, chiropractic philosophy seems an anachronism. How can chiropractic principles be taken seriously when the scientific world has achieved such technological miracles? These miracles have been the result of an ever increasing pool of knowledge relative to the human body. Scientific knowledge has improved so much that it overshadows the other aspects of clinical practice. The result is a reversal of the manner in which chiropractors were originally taught. The scientific information that was once limited has now expanded, so more time and effort is directed toward these subjects. As attention has been diverted to science, the principles of chiropractic are not studied as extensively as in the past. The world has changed since the time chiropractic was founded and its principles formulated. Technologically, the healing arts have advanced, but in terms of health there have been no significant improvements in the way sick people are treated.

The unfortunate truth is that increased knowledge has caused patients to be viewed as tissue, an organism that will respond to a variety of therapies. The techniques used in treating the sick have improved, but have the results? The healing arts may improve the quantity of time a patient may experience, but what has been the healing arts' contribution to the quality of life? This fact is supported by statistical evidence that the health of individuals has not really improved. On a non-statistical basis, it can be seen that the quality of life most people experience is below their expectations.

Each day, since prehistoric time, the sun rises in the morning and sets in the evening. The sun accomplishes this feat without the help of man, although man can share in the wonder of this sequence by observing it. With all our scientific knowledge, man has been unable to improve upon this sequence. The principles of chiropractic are similar to the rising and setting of the sun. They are a reflection of things natural that have become stronger with time. These principles are the foundation of each and every chiropractor' s office. They hold the same veracity today as when they were first formulated. Though they might gain more credibility and acceptance with each new fact we learn regarding all aspects of life, the basic principles remain the same.

Of the thirty-three principles that have been defined there are six which hold specific clinical relevance. These are the principles which should be omnipresent whenever a chiropractor treats a patient. It seems though, that all chiropractic principles have been removed from our clinical approach to patients.

There are many reasons for the writing of this book. I have been privileged to be affiliated with chiropractic for the past fifteen years, first as a patient, then as a student, and now as a practicing chiropractor. I have watched on the sidelines as chiropractic has become a visible force in healing. Now, having been both a student and teacher, I find the "new breed" of chiropractic student, while more scientifically oriented, to be philosophically deficient. Chiropractic, it must be re-emphasized, is a science, and an art and philosophy, yet the art and philosophy have seemingly been sacrificed in imitation of the scientific emphasis of allopathic education. One reason is to bridge the gap between the strictly scientific approach to patients with the principles of chiropractic that have apparently become neglected in clinical practice.

Chiropractic is on the threshold of becoming the most prominent branch of the healing arts. This goal will be realized by effectively treating sick patients and taking steps to re-educate a chiropractically ignorant society. History has been distorted to a point where the public believes chiropractic has followed allopathic medicine in sequence. This is not true. The ideas of Hippocrates have always been associated with the allopath, but are actually more compatible to the holistic concept of chiropractic. The difference in health attitudes did not start with the controversy between the allopath and the chiropractor, but dates far back into antiquity. A second reason is to put into perspective the history of healing. The events that have contributed to our current beliefs regarding health are not generally known. Although this text is not an exhaustive history of the subject, it does bring some facts to light.

The direction that healing has taken in this country was determined some time ago. All branches of the healing arts have taken measures to help satisfy the needs of the public. Although these steps were taken with the best intentions, some mistakes are evident. Chiropractic can only be responsible for correcting those mistakes it has committed. It has a further responsibility to learn from the mistakes of other professions to insure steering clear of any other pitfalls. If these objectives are attained chiropractic will strengthen its position as a viable alternative to traditional medicine. If any of the ideas contained within the book can contribute to the continued growth of chiropractic, it will have served a valuable purpose.

The future of chiropractic is based on the ability to understand chiropractic principles as an "old fashioned" chiropractor does, and enhance the efficacy and application of those principles with a thorough knowledge of the contemporary ideas of anatomy, physiology, and biomechanics. Combining science with art and based on a sound philosophy, the way chiropractic was originally proposed, chiropractors will facilitate the healing of patients and insure the success of chiropractic.

"THE ONLY LIMIT TO OUR REALIZATION OF TOMORROW WILL BE OUR DOUBTS OF TODAY."

CHAPTER 1

"Every profession is a conspiracy against the laity."
George Bernard Shaw

The concept that nature is smarter than man is not new, nor did it originate with chiropractic. The controversy that erupted in 1895, when D.D. Palmer discovered chiropractic, was an age old controversy that was really spawned in ancient Greece. In truth the problem started long before that, but in ancient Greece the battle lines were drawn, and these are still in effect today.

The exact origin of therapeutic manipulation has never been determined. It is known, however, that prehistoric man practiced some form of spinal adjustment. This is evidenced by cave drawings circa 17,500 B.C., that were uncovered in France. Ancient manuscripts contain concise descriptions of chiropractic type treatment. The Kong Fou document, written about 2700 B.C. gives some advice on tissue manipulation. The Chinese have, for centuries, employed the method of rubbing the bones of the neck to relieve a variety of ailments. They also applied pressure with a copper coin in this region to ease ailments of the nerves.

An ancient Egyptian papyrus, dated 1700 B.C. also lends evidence that spinal manipulation was performed. Egyptian rock carvings made centuries ago show healers placing their hands along the spinal column. Greek papyri, circa 1500 B.C., gave instructions on the treatment of low back conditions. Other diverse cultures from around the globe also practiced some form of manipulation; among them are Japanese, Indians of Asia, Egyptians, Babylonians, Syrians, Hindus, Tibetans, Tahitians and the Incas of South America. The endurance of North American Indians is attributed to the care given by the squaw mother who binds the little papoose to a board until its spine assumes the primary curves essential to proper development.

There are also certain allopathic practices that have been recorded in ancient history. There are accounts of Egyptian physicians being specialists in only one part of the body or one disease. Egyptians also compounded drugs, embalmed and did surgery, in addition to utilizing manipulation in their treatment of the sick. The practice of defensive medicine also has its roots in ancient Egypt. There, cures were revealed by the gods and codified by Thoth. If a patient died as a result of a physician deviating from the book of Thoth, the act was considered a capital crime. Society has become more civilized. Now when a doctor is found to be negligent in his treatment of a patient, a different standard is used to determine the penalty exacted.

Other modern medical practices are documented in history. In early civilizations, doctors were regarded as of a high social class. They spoke with authority in an uncommon language, disguised their secret methods in occult studies and frequently used fear to motivate patients to accept their prescriptions. Perhaps practices such as these inspired the quotation that begins this chapter. To a degree these practices are still in effect today. However, they are no longer readily accepted by the public. Instead, patient consciousness regarding health has been raised and more and more patients want to know what kind of treatment they are receiving and how it works.

The different viewpoints in the healing arts today have many roots in history. In some primitive societies it was believed that the cause of disease could be found in some outside influence that entered the victim. Thus rose the belief in hexes, evil forces and demons. Some societies even thought to blame afflictions on the will of the gods. Epilepsy, at one time, was known as the sacred disease. In modern terminology, the belief that germs cause disease can be traced to this notion.

Other societies looked upon disease as an abstraction of the soul from its body. If, in fact, the soul was within a person, and was the very essence of the person's individuality, an alteration of the soul would cause disease. This point of view is presently defined by the concept that subluxation causes disease.

From these two general points of view, evolved the various theories that supported the "within" and "without" philosophies. The conflict has been passed down through the ages. It is still a point of contention among today's health care practitioners. At this point it should be noted that there is an intermingling of fact and fiction in the roots of healing. Much of what has been passed down historically is a mixture of science and religion. In a simple world, men looked for simple answers to explain the complex questions and phenomena they could not understand. They found their answers in the gods. Through the actions of the gods men were able to understand the wonders of the universe. By understanding the nature of some of the gods, a pattern of thought that has determined our attitudes regarding health could develop. Although the roots of healing and the inherent philosophical differences are prehistoric, there is a definite starting point to the conflict. Two Greek deities, Hygeia and Asclepius, by their very natures, represent the difference in health care attitudes.

The goddess Hygeia watched over the health of Athens. She was identified with Athena, the goddess of reason. Although Hygeia was associated with health, she was not actually involved in treating the sick. Instead, she was the guardian of health who symbolized the belief that men could remain well if they lived according to reason.

According to Greek legend, Asclepius was the first physician. He was the son of Apollo and the nymph Coronis, and was taught the art of healing by the centaur Chiron. He gained fame by mastering the curative powers of plants, as well as ability with the use of his knife. His fame was so great that he eventually ascended to the position as the god of medicine.

In ancient sculpture, Asclepius is seen standing, dressed in a long cloak, with a bare breast. His usual attribute is a clublike staff with a serpent coiled around it. This staff, with its single serpent is the only true symbol of medicine. The caduceus, with its winged staff and intertwined serpents, which is frequently used in this country to represent traditional medicine, is without medical relevance since it truly represents the magic wand of Hermes or Mercury, the messenger of the gods and patron of trade.

Because of Asclepius' powers, Hygeia was relegated to a subservient role in his retinue, most probably as his daughter. Here she was joined by her sister Panakeia, who because of her knowledge of drugs from plants and the earth, became omnipotent as a healing goddess.

The unification of both deities seemed to take place in the person of Hippocrates. For Hippocrates, rational living and fitness to the environment were essential tenets of his health care philosophy. He complimented this philosophy with the clinical application of mild remedies to assist nature in the healing of the sick. During his lifetime, in addition to his views, there were two other schools of thought.

There existed priest doctors, dedicated to the god of medicine and the serpent cult. These doctors based their treatments upon bathing, fasting, drugs and suggestion. They also performed surgery under the influence of sleeping potions and hypnotic suggestion.

Hippocrates served as chief physician and teacher at the Coan school, located on the island of Cos. To Hippocrates, disease was not the ravages of an indwelling demon, but instead, a condition of disharmony in a person's body. A battle between the disease and the self healing tendency of the body, the vis medicae naturae. Hippocrates believed that the sick body triggers natural forces to restore equilibrium and restore good health.

Hippocrates founded his teachings on the firm belief that, while the cause of disease could be found either outside or inside the victim, "it is our natures that are the physicians or our diseases.'' The knowledge of his time was limited; therefore, the corrective mechanisms were not known, but the basic idea was understood. It should be noted that at this time neither the thermometer nor the stethescope had been invented. The more advanced diagnostic equipment employed today had not yet been developed. Despite this, Hippocrates proved to be an unparalleled diagnostician. To achieve this diagnostic acumen, Hippocrates utilized his powers of observation and logical reasoning. Writing of epilepsy, which was then known as a sacred disease he said, "it is no more sacred than any other disease, but has a natural cause and its supposed divine origin is due to man's inexperience.'' He had an uncanny ability to foretell the course of a malady, laying more stress on prognosis than diagnosis. Therefore, the emphasis of treatment at the Coan school was on the patient.

Implicit in his writings is that both health and disease are under control of natural laws and reflect the influence exerted by the environment and the way of life. In one of his works, "Air, Water, Places," which today would be classified as a treatise on ecology, he noted the effect of food, occupation and especially of climate, in causing disease. In aphorisms he reminded his students not to meddle with, nor hinder, r-*ure's attempt toward recovery. Hippocrates himself usually confined his treatment to assisting nature with mild remedies. Once the treatment was administered, the patient, through his physiology, reacted in his own individual way against the disease. Therefore, health depended on a state of equilibrium among the various internal factors which govern the operations of the body and the mind. This equilibrium is reached only when man lives in harmony with his external environment.

If both health and disease were under the control of natural laws and health is the preferred state, disease is an infringement upon natural laws. Time and again, Hippocrates stated the concept that the life and lifestyle of the patient were implicated in the disease process and that the cause is to be found in the combination of circumstances rather than in the simple direct effect of some external agency. Hippocrates was a proponent of rational living, a point of view that links him with Hygeia. He believed that disease would ensue when changes in conditions are too rapid and too violent to allow the adaptive mechanisms to come into play. Changes that occur whether they be seasonal or environmental, are best when they are done moderately and gradually. This Hippocratic view is as true and accurate today as when it was first espoused. Any profound change in social patterns will influence the health of nations and the incidence of disease in their populations. The sickness of an individual is not easily separated from the sickness of society. In our lifetime, perhaps the best example to support this point of view can be found in the Viet Nam war. Can anyone deny that the stresses and frustrations caused by this debacle contributed to illness in this country?

The health of populations is affected not only by medical practices employed in any given era, but also from social, technical and economic factors. What will be the effect of women's liberation or the refinement of food products or economic recessions and depressions? Only time will lend a clue as to what effect society will endure in terms of sickness and disease as a response to these changes.

Hippocrates believed that every practitioner of medicine, "was to be skilled in nature and strive to know what man is in relation to food, drink and occupation, and what effect each of these has on the other." He also recognized the importance of the spine and spinal manipulation. He said, "Get knowledge of the spine for it is the requisite for many diseases."

The other school of thought that existed in this time period was the Cnidian school. This school had been influenced by Egyptian and Mesopotamian cultures and emphasized the treatment of the disease rather than the patient. Euryphon was the chief physician and teacher. As Hippocrates had influenced the Coan school, so too did Euryphon influence the Cnidian attitudes toward treatment. The Cnidian physicians aimed at exact diagnosis, classification and specific therapy. A broad spectrum approach that emphasized lifestyle and environment as affecting a patient's health was inconsistent with his belief. Euryphon believed that definite events occurred which affected an individual. These events, once directed towards an individual, transformed a healthy person to a sick patient. Euryphon's approach promoted a specific cause for each disease. He felt the Hippocratic approach was too philosophical compared to his more practical method.

Other great healers gained fame because of their ability to treat the sick, and as such, have influenced patient care to this day. Herodicus, the first great drugless healer, achieved wide fame in curing diseases by correcting abnormalities of the spine. He refrained from using drugs and tonics and utilized manual manipulation and therapeutic exercise in treating his patients.

Serapion taught a timeless lesson to all students of healing, past and present. There are no two patients alike, and because of this, we must depend on experience alone in our treatment of the sick. Anatomy, physiology and pathology might deviate from those standards taught students of healing. Therefore, in treating patients, the best method is combining book knowledge with the intuition that is guided by observation. This skill is inborn, but needs experience and practice to make it functional.

After Hippocrates the most distinguished physician of antiqquity was Galen, the founder of experimental physiology. Despite the limited resources of accumulated knowledge, his anatomical investigations are complete and accurate. He dissected apes and lower animals, describing what he saw and attempting to relate his findings to human anatomy.

Among other things, Galen taught the proper position and relations of the vertebrae and the spinal column. He advised his students, "Look to the nervous system as the key to maximum health." This statement is perhaps based on his studies where he sectioned the spinal cord at various levels and observed the resulting sensory and motor disturbance.

He describes the heart and its three layers of fibers, although he hesitated to call the tissues muscle. This reluctance was due to his observation that heart muscle was characteristically different from other, ordinary muscle. He also recorded that section of its nerve supply was not followed by cessation of its activities.

The founder of experimental physiology also had a philosophical side to him. Galen was a firm believer in a supreme creator of the universe in all its parts. He claimed that God's purpose could be elicited in great detail from examination of His work. To this end he set himself to prove that the bodily organs are in such perfect relation to the functions to which they minister, that it is impossible to imagine any better arrangement.

Galen was a tremendous teacher who achieved wide fame in the field of medical education. He knew of insensible perspiration. He ligatured the recurrent laryngeal nerve. He espoused the examination of urine in certain diseases, the value of specific foods, critical days in fever, the significance of the pulse, the character of the arteries and the nature of parasitic worms.

There have been other physicians and teachers who contributed to health history. Many of the accomplishments of these people have been improved upon by the technological advances that have since occurred, but this brief history illustrates the origins of health attitudes and the basic differences that pervade the healing arts. The controversy is deep rooted in history, yet as contemporary as each new day. The broad spectrum approach maintains there is a correlation between the state of one's health and environmental factors. The specific etiology theory maintains there is a specific cause that creates a disease condition. The difference in the two is underscored by the lack of resolve that has lingered through the ages. From Hygeia and Asclepius, to Hippocrates and Euryphon, to the chiropractor and the allopathic physician, the controversy has never changed. On the one hand there is an attempt by man to control nature by living within its confines reasonably, while on the other hand, there is the attempt to control nature by the imposition of pills, potents and surgery.

"I NOT ONLY USE ALL THE BRAINS I HAVE BUT ALL I CAN BORROW."

—*WOODROW WILSON*

CHAPTER 2

Modern chiropractic is in a unique position. It finds itself compelled to maintain the principles and philosophy that have enabled it to become the largest, drugless healing profession in the world: yet, it must remain contemporary in thought to effectively treat those patients in need of chiropractic care. The dilemma that confronts chiropractic is: How can chiropractors be successful in the twentieth century, utilizing principles that seem, to say the least, outdated? How can sophisticated human beings accept the principles and practices of healing the sick that have been passed down through the ages? The reason chiropractors can apply such dated principles is that they have endured and consistently achieved more results than any modern wonder drug. Each year new pills and drugs are put on the market in a seemingly endless parade of futility. Yet, the principles that have maintained the chiropractic profession have remained unaltered. Why? Because they are true to the tenets of nature and the rational approach in treating the sick.

The chiropractic profession has grown since 1895, but a large segment of the population is still ignorant of the concept of health and the services provided by chiropractors. This ignorance is a reflection of the health attitudes that have been pushed on society by the medical establishment and the pharmaceutical industry. There are daily advertisements on television, in magazines and newspapers that promote the use of medication to relieve the suffering of the multitudes. The result is that more and more members of society depend on drugs and doctors for meeting the ordinary problems of everyday life.

An adjunctive movement that downplays individuality and undermines personal ability is produced by the advertisements of a variety of products. According to these advertisements, in order to be attractive or desirable one must wear a certain brand of clothes or cologne. These same ads infer that if if were not for the use of toothpaste or breath mints there would be no relationships between men and women. It seems society is programmed on all levels to accept outside assistance in order to achieve any kind of well being.

The medical establishment, which has long criticized the chiropractic profession for being unscientific and too philosophical, labors under the pretense that being scientific and aphilosophical, yields better clinical results. In general, this is not true. In this lifetime, one in four members of society will have to undergo some form of psychotherapy. Life expectancy past the age of forty has not significantly increased in several decades, and the quality of life, due to stress and frustration, is questionable. Each year a larger portion of income is spent on medical care and the quest for health. These facts have not only been accepted as a way of life, but people continually contribute to their growth by insisting on living in a way incompatible with overall health.

The spell that has been cast on society by traditional medicine is awesome. It has been and continues to be reinforced on a daily basis, and with each passing day, the power of traditional medicine grows. In truth, the power of a doctor is based neither on science, as some would have us believe, nor on philosophy, but on faith. A doctor, any doctor, is the personification of the intelligence and skill that unites a patient with health. Because these qualities are possessed by those individuals trained in schools of healing, patients must have faith in their doctors. This kind of faith is reminiscent of ancient times when doctors were considered elite members of a priesthood. Allopathic physicians produce new therapies and surgical feats, disguise their alterations of established procedures in mystical and impressive language, then wait for the recognition and accolades of the masses. Chiropractors, in their effort to survive, have been overwhelmed by the deluge of medical propaganda. They, too, can be accused of utilizing mystical power, although for a different reason. There is not enough patient education on an individual basis to allow access to the knowledge essential to their health. Because of this, effort should be made to effectively counteract the large scale public relations that promote the allopathic point of view. The best public relations for any chiropractor is a patient who has responded favorably to treatment. If, in the course of treatment, the patient has been educated about chiropractic, he will become health conscious. This awareness will enable the patient to be sensitive to his own needs, as well as the health requirements for the other people in his life. A skeptical person who feels he might benefit from chiropractic care will be more comforted by a satisfied patient who can share a personal experience of chiropractic rather than any form of media advertising.

Sensationalistic advertising, which has become a common method of exposing the public to chiropractic, cheapens the profession and falls short of educating patients. An occasional lecture does not fortify the concept of rational living and the necessity of chiropractic care. Chiropractors have always been credited with being able to relate to and speak with patients. This process of communication is essential to the growth of chiropractic. Unfortunately, the current trend seems to be similar to the allopathic aproach: administer treatment and forget about communicating with patients.

People can accept the limitations of their physical ability. They cannot accept the limitations of society. Newspapers are packed with stories about the atrocities of modern civilization. There are stories about war, murder, rape, poverty. People live in the land of freedom and opportunity, yet their thoughts are always directed toward the disagreeable events of life. Knowledge of these situations is detrimental to an individual's health. Even more detrimental is the accompanying frustration that is caused by being unable to change these situations. Why should a patient be well to live in a society that is sick?

The problems of society are caused by people. A doctor cannot cure the ills of society by treating society. A doctor can only be responsible for utilizing his skills in the best interest of his patients. This is the focus of a true healer. A true healer treats patients on an individual basis, providing them with the opportunity to achieve health. When this is achieved, their health is a reflection of their lives, and in this way, they can more fully contribute to society.

How is it that society pursues health through faith in drugs and science, while alternate forms of healing are looked upon with scorn and ridicule? There are several factors that directly influenced this present state of affairs.

The American public has been led to believe the "breakthroughs" that have occurred in science have been the key to achieving the high standard of health enjoyed in this country. The life expectancy in some European countries that do not have the benefits of living in such an advanced society, is greater than our own. The American citizen is encouraged to believe that money can create drugs for the cure of heart disease, cancer and mental disease. Consider the number of telethons and the increased media coverage given these projects. There is insufficient effort made to recognize the factors that contribute to the high incidence of these conditions. There is even less effort made to control the indiscretions of our everyday life so as to limit the occurrence of such conditions. Perhaps these conditions, which are directly linked to the irresponsibility of patients, are caused by their orientation regarding health. This irresponsibility can best be described as blind faith.

The blind faith factor has caused intelligent people to believe what allopathic doctors say regarding their health. This same faith that elevates doctors above the status of mere mortals is also given to the magic of drugs. Why monitor one's health if it can easily be restored with the application of some magic tonic? Often, the word miracle is attributed to the effect of a new drug. This new found miracle then becomes the source of comfort and hope to the masses. There are few individuals who understand how the miracle drug might work. Even fewer know of its side effects, but as long as some fantastic attribute is attached to the drug, people believe. Thus, the sophistication that society pretends to possess is as illusory as the curative power of the drugs they seek. Men still find it easier to believe in miracles and mysterious forces rather than trust in rational processess. Men today want miracles just as much as in the past. Although it is true that faith in the healing power of ancient gods has decreased, faith still maintains more power than reason in human beings.

Aside from the oath that bears reference to his name, most people know nothing of Hippocrates. They do not know he was a physician of considerable skill, able to achieve remarkable results with his patients long before the modern scientific era. By empirically manipulating the psychological, physiological and, social factors that affected a person's health, he achieved the reputation as the greatest healer of antiquity. His observations and writings are the cornerstone of healing. He possessed keen insight into the human condition and transformed his thoughts into timeless writings that have been passed down through the ages. Most people regard the fame of Hippocrates as his affiliation with traditional medicine. They do not realize that, more than anything else, Hippocrates represents a concept in healing. The concept that man must live in harmony with his environment, and when in a state of disharmony, the physician is to intervene in the most natural way. Yet this tradition has been obscured in the last century. It is consistent with the chiropractic concept of health, but seemingly in opposition to the germ theory and limited causality concept of scientific medicine.

Harmony with nature and within ourselves is an intuitively attractive idea. To live in accordance with the natural forces of life and in harmony with one's environment has been a recurring philosphical theme. Today, this quest has been all but forgotten as most people find it easier to achieve health by depending on doctors and outside agents, rather than attempting to live wisely.

There are examples of entire cultures which have pursued health by following their natural instincts. Oriental and holistic practitioners treat the imbalance and allow the body to heal itself from within. The focus of these practitioners is not the disease. Instead, the focus is the patient as he is related to society, the environment, and himself. These healers benefit from the fact that their practices are a combination of a philosophy and of clinical experience. The Oriental is mindful of the yin and yang, the balance and harmony of nature. The holistic healer maintains an intuitive clinical sense and a deep respect for the natural healing power of the body, as it relates to all environmental factors. The drawbacks to these alien approaches is that they are incongruous with the attitude of today's society. Man today has time to do all things but heal himself. He will allow investments time to yield a profit, he will allow young athletes time to reach their athletic potential, he will allow time for everything else but his homeostatic mechanisms to synchronize with his lifestyle.

Enter traditional medicine. The benefit of traditional medicine is that it buys time by treating the disease. If in the time bought from medicine the imbalance that is the source of the disease is not corrected, sickness will occur again. The unfortunate side effect of this transitory feeling of health is that not only does it afford the time to find the source of the disease, it also enables the individual to get back into the routine that has contributed to this decline in health. Regardless, health has been restored and fate has been sidestepped. Society continues to live this illusion. Pain, a by product of disease, is a reminder there is an imbalance in our lives. The end result of life is death, but this is nothing more than a natural cycle that has been established for centuries. The important aspect of this cycle is not that we die, but rather, the quality of the life we live. This is the focus of a true healer, treating patients on an individual basis, so their health is a reflection of their lives, and in this way, they can more fully contribute to society.

Traditional medicine does not maintain the approach just discussed, yet it is the most dominant branch of the healing arts. Again we are faced with the question, why? The answer is not easily discerned, nor is it confined to one field of learning. The answer has its roots in philosophy, its cause in sociology, and its effect in the distortion of the truth.

At one time man was considered a noble savage. The ideal life was maintained by living in harmony with nature. This harmony was, and still is, the pursuit of many people.

As man and civilization "advanced", the needs of society were expanding at a tremendous rate. The need to mechanize the processess of manufacturing gave birth to one of the most significant movements in the history of man, the industrial revolution. The effects of this revolution spread, at first, throughout Europe, but eventually through the entire world.

England prospered through the technological advances that characterized the movement, but it also suffered its ill side effects that manifested themselves in the destruction of human values. In time it became obvious that disease and physical frailty were most common among the poor classes. The poor populations of manufacturing towns became infested with disease. Now the quest for happiness was no longer a life of harmony with nature, but instead, survival. Since the factors that accompanied disease were always the same; want, dirt, and pollution, it was believed that health could be restored by bringing back to the multitudes pure air, pure water, pure food and pleasant surroundings. With this in mind, civic organizations undertook the task of health restoration. Their common sense approach was successful and the quality of life, and health, of the English working class was greatly improved. Oddly enough, as the quality of life increased, the disease rate decreased.

Munich, Germany, experienced a significant decrease in the incidence of typhoid that is directly attributed to having water brought into the city from the surrounding mountains and having the city sewage diluted. Anti-filth campaigns were waged in Spain during the early part of the nineteenth century, the result being that Barcelona did not experience any further outbreaks of yellow fever.

Perhaps the best example of the multi-causal origin of diseases could best be found in the case of the renowned scientist, Rudolph Virchow. He was appointed to study an epidemic that was raging through the industrial district of Upper Silesia. In a minority report, Virchow traced the origin of the epidemic to unfavorable meterological conditions! A famine had occurred because heavy rains had ruined the year's crops. Furthermore, the following winter had been extremely severe, forcing the poor to huddle together in their homes, cold and hungry. It was then a typhus epidemic had broken out, first spreading through the poor population, and eventually reaching the wealthier class. From this experience, Virchow proposed the theory that poverty is the breeder of disease and that it was the responsibility of the physician to support social reforms that would reconstruct society in a pattern more favorable to the health of man. According to Virchow, the treatment of individual cases is only a small aspect of medicine. More important is the control of crowd disease, which demand social, and possibly political action.

There is also evidence to indicate that a certain amount of natural resistance has been established and has contributed to the control of disease and infection. The mortality rate in North America and Europe from tuberculosis has been steadily on the decline since the turn of the 19th century. No drug therapy was available during this time, vaccination was not practiced, and those therapeutic procedures available were of limited value and reached only a small percentage of the population.

The same holds true for measles. The incidence of measles was on the decline before the measles vaccine was introduced. Statistical evidence confirms the disease is much less a problem today then it was several years ago. This decrease has been attributed to the measles vaccine, while the decreased incidence of measles should really be credited to man's natural resistance. The body will build natural immunity to a disease process if it is exposed to the disease over a period of time.

Because the decrease in the death rate appeared obvious to everyone after 1900, scientific medicine and the germ theory in particular have been given all the credit for all the improvement of the general health of the public. This is an injustice. An even greater injustice is the present day belief that the control of diseases can be attributed to the widespread use of antibacterial drugs. In truth, the mortality of many infections had begun to recede in Europe and North America long before the specific methods of therapy were introduced and the germ theory of disease was a popular concept.

This is not to negate the positive contributions science and medicine have made to the health of mankind. Scientific medicine has greatly helped deal with the negative side effects of urban and industrial civilization.

Louis Pasteur, one of the most renowned scientists of all time, was able to influence society on many planes due to his varied scientific accomplishments. He disproved the theory of spontaneous generation. He proved that microorganisms cause fermentation and disease; he originated and was the first to use vaccines for chicken pox, cholera, anthrax, and rabies. Through his work he was also able to save the wine and silk industries of France. When Pasteur proposed his germ theory of disease, he did not envision a simple connection between germs and disease. He was cognizant that other factors also contributed to the occurrence of a disease process. The simplistic outlook has been the result of a lack of education on the part of patients and their miseducation by physicians. The oversimplification is: germs cause disease; to treat the disease, kill germs by using drugs.

Some medical breakthroughs were the result of plain old common sense combined with an acute sense of observation.

Ignaz Semmelweis, a Hungarian obstetrician, noted that the death rate seemed to be higher in certain clinics where the medical students and physicians came directly to the ward from the morgue or autopsy rooms. Upon witnessing the autopsy of a pathologist who had died of an infectious process that developed after a dissection wound, he observed and noted the pathological changes that had occurred as a result of the infection were similar to those of a woman who had died of puerperal fever. Semmelweis concluded the infectious nature of puerperal fever and instituted certain practices intended to prevent the spread of infection. On the wards he supervised, all hands had to be cleaned before a patient was examined and the rooms had to be regularly cleaned. The result was the mortality in his service immediately dropped. He published his views, but they were met with strong opposition by the medical establishment.

Joseph Lord Lister noted the similarity between wound infections and certain fermentative and putrefactive changes, which Pasteur had already proved were caused by microorganisms. He concluded that wound infections were caused by microbes. With this in mind, he started protecting wounds with dressings saturated with a solution of phenol. He also developed operating room procedures calculated to destroy microorganisms.

Scientific medicine, combining the works of Pasteur, and the observations of Semmelweis and Lister, have been able to produce some preventative measures against disease. There have been other medical accomplishments that are a credit to the medical profession and a definite boon to the health of man, but to credit medicine with stemming the tide of infectious disease during the past century is wrong. By the time scientists entered the battle at the beginning of the twentieth century, social reformers had already reduced the effects of poor nutrition and infectious disease. As Rene DuBos, an eminent scientist, has pointed out, the introduction of easy to launder, inexpensive cotton undergarments and transparent glass that brought light into the most humble dwelling have contributed more to the control of infection than all the drugs and medical practices combined. The accolades given scientific medicine in its control of infectious disease should really be shared with social reformers whose efforts laid the groundwork for the overall improvement of health experienced by man. The trends of improvement extend throughout history. It has been established in society by reformers, and medical science has not significantly altered them.

The public should be informed about the events that have helped shape the currently accepted beliefs regarding health. The public should be made aware of the chiropractic concept of health. They must be made to realize that the breakthroughs that have influenced the health of society have not been achieved through the work of science alone.

Medical research continues its attempts at finding the causes of a myriad of diseases. With all the research that is taking place in laboratories, few have been looking at our society or environment. There has never been a prescription written to provide relief for a patient suffering from poverty, decaying housing, or social alienation. However, these problems are rarely addressed as being causal factors in disease. As a society we are overfed and undernourished. We eat to excess, drink to excess and overindulge. We work and play at a staggering rate, yet there is a residual frustration in our lives. No longer are we obsessed with death and disease. Man has become civilized to a point where threats of physical danger no longer exist, nutritional deficiencies are a thing of the past and disease has been held in check by medical science. The newest threats come in the form of vascular disease, cancer, and mental disease. The unfortunate fact is that today, we must deal not only with those diseases caused by our lifestyles, but we have yet to conquer the diseases of days gone by. Because people have been made to believe the best way to safeguard their health is to support the development of new drugs, they have lost their instinct for health. There is overwhelming evidence that our most prevalent diseases are directly related to our lifestyles, but still the rational approach to health is held in deference to the long awaited medical miracle. Modern medical science has proven itself inadequate in treating its patients. The public, many of whom have had some bad experience with an allopath, is aware of the problem and is actively searching for a viable alternative to traditional medicine. Now with proper re-education and competent, ethical care chiropractors can prove to the public that such an alternative does exist. The chiropractic profession, long the second class citizen of the healing arts, can now take its place as the leader in the field of health.

CHAPTER 3

The misconceptions regarding health have been transmitted to attitudes concerning doctors. For instance, consider the definition of the word doctor, from the Latin root meaning teacher. Rare today is the doctor who will instruct patients about the maintenance of their health. Dorland's Medical Dictionary defines a doctor as a practitioner of the healing arts; one who has received a degree from a college of medicine, osteopathy or veterinary medicine, licensed to practice by a state.

Another example of our altered conception can be seen by looking at the word physician. It is derived from the Greek word meaning nature, yet nowhere in the modern interpretation of physician is there any reference made toward nature. To Hippocrates, every practitioner of medicine, "was to be skilled in nature and must know what man is in relation to food, drink and occupation, and what effect each of these has on the other."

Today, Dorland's Medical Dictionary defines a physician as follows: an authorized practitioner of medicine, as one graduated from a college of medicine or osteopathy and licensed by the appropriate state board. The focus of a physician is no longer geared towards clinical ability, but rather, the recognition of the appropriate societal authorities.

Because of the defensive posture assumed by most doctors, no longer is there a correlation between daily activities and interactions of patients with an effective treatment plan intended to help the patient in the most holistic manner. Instead, doctors recommend advice only as it relates to their specialty. No longer is the compassionate treatment of the sick the primary concern of the physician. Seemingly, the primary concern is the establishment and maintenance of a reputation.

In view of the distortion one can establish by looking at the words doctor and physician, let us examine the word medicine. According to Dorland's Medical Dictionary, medicine is: any drug or remedy; the art and science of the diagnosis and treatment of disease and the maintenance of health; the treatment of disease by other than surgical means. The definition of remedy is: anything that cures, palliates or prevents disease.

The definition of allopathy is: a term applied to that system of therapeutics in which diseases are treated by producing a condition incompatible with or antagonistic to the condition to be cured or alleviated. One of the more interesting definitions is assigned to surgery, which is: that branch of medicine which treats diseases, injuries and deformities by manual or operative methods. The roots of the word surgeon are from the Greek words CHEIR meaning hand, and ERGON meaning work. It seems that by definition, the focus of a chiropractor and a surgeon are similar, the difference lies in their clinical orientation.

The following definition of chiropractic is a combination of the thoughts of two great pioneer chiropractors, B.J. Palmer and Willard Carver.

Chiropractic is a philosophy, science and art. It is the science that teaches health in anatomical relation and disease in disrelation. It is the philosophy of things natural, and the art of adjusting the segments of the spine by hand, for the correction of disease.

It is amazing how the term medicine has become synonymous with the allopathic physician. It is clear, by definition, that chiropractic can be considered medicine. It is even more clear, by clinical results, that chiropractors practice medicine in its purest form. Although chiropractic is not, nor ever will be, associated with drug therapy, it is a remedy. It is also a distinct art and science which employs diagnosis as an indicator of how a patient might best be treated, whether exclusively within the realm of chiropractic, or by another branch of the healing arts. Chiropractors, acting in the best interest of their patients, should never forget the ancient law of healing, i.e., "Salus aegroti suprema lex" the welfare of the ailing is the supreme law. Adherence to such a mandate can only be achieved when one is secure in the belief in his abilities and the principles of his profession. It is obvious that there are not enough referrals from our allopathic counterparts. They have taken such a radical anti-chiropractic position in the past, and are so ignorant of the services performed by chiropractors, that they call ill afford to allow us the opportunity to succeed where they have failed. In this regard they would do well to follow the advice of the noted physician John Mennell: "...under certain circumstances I think you are justified in asking a well trained manipulator, whoever he might be, to treat your patient for that specific complaint, just as you would ask a pharmacist to make up a prescription...Do not deprive your patients of relief from pain because of your prejudice."

The definition of chiropractic on the preceeding page covers the spectrum of what chiropractic is. It is the combined effort of the ideas of two men, who in their own ways, shaped the future of chiropractic. Their legacy is an emerging profession that must unify its efforts in order to prevail. This unification can begin by acknowledging that, despite our education interpretation, the principles of chiropractic are the same for all chiropractors.

Society has imposed certain restrictions on the chiropractic profession. Each state has its own rules and regulations regarding the scope of practice allowed chiropractors. The blame for such a situation existing rests not with chiropractic, but with chiropractors.

From the beginning, chiropractic has been a controversial profession. The different points of view that existed among early chiropractors lingers to this very day. The differences are not clinical or philosophical, but really seem to be egotistical in nature. The quality of a chiropractor was determined by whose policies the chiropractor adhered to, not by his ability to treat the sick. Just as the chiropractic pioneers were unable to blend their differences to form a strong, unified profession, today's chiropractors are equally unwilling. It seems ludicrous to maintain differences that are based upon egotism when the principles of the profession are the same for all chiropractors.

If chiropractic is to advance, unity is essential. Chiropractors should apply their principles to the condition of the profession. The healing power of the body comes from within the body. The chiropractic profession must heal itself from within the ranks of chiropractors. The common bond, chiropractic principles, is alive and well and helping sick people get well. It is time for the profession to get well.

There are a variety of techniques available to chiropractors. It is up to the individual doctor to decide which analysis and techniques he can comfortably use. It is up to the individual chiropractor to decide the parameters within which he can comfortably and effectively practice chiropractic. There must be a mutual respect between chiropractors. There is no need for animosity within the profession when the profession must endure adversity from outside sources.

Chiropractic is a concept that supercedes the bias of individual chiropractors. Chiropractic will endure, not only because of the efforts of chiropractors, but also, in spite of them.

A cure can be effected only at the prerogative of nature. Each individual has the potential to heal, but whether or not this potential is realized is the result of the doctor's skill at facilitating the healing process and the body's willingness to respond. Whether the doctor be a chiropractor, allopath, osteopath or surgeon, the ultimate healing ability still rests with the patient.

CHAPTER 4

The chiropractic profession has received certain benefits from its relationship with the allopathic profession. Due to the prominent position traditional medicine has maintained in society, the education of medical doctors was more scrutinized than any other branch of the healing arts. During the eighteenth and nineteenth centuries, almost any man in America could become a doctor if he could afford the tuition fees or had family contacts for arranging to serve as an apprentice to an established practitioner. Not even a high school education was needed and it was possible to become a doctor in six months of study. Through the years, the conditions• that have determined the future of healing have been altered. In 1910, a relatively unknown high school teacher named Alexander Flexnor published Bulletin #4 for the Carnegie Foundation for the Advancement of Teaching titled, "Medical Education in the United States and Canada". The effect was the revolution of medical education. From this point on, the emphasis would be on medicine as a science, while the practice of the art would be relegated to a secondary role.

The immediate impact of the Flexnor report was to close many of the substandard medical schools of the day, leaving the field to those better equipped, staffed and organized. Overproduction of poorly trained and ill educated physicians was sharply curtailed and standards of medical licensure and practice improved. The long term effect of this report and the ensuing battle over which direction the education of medical doctors would go, has produced highly trained technicians, many of whom do not exhibit the sensitivity or compassion to be called doctors.

In truth, Flexnor won his battle to standardize medical education and improve the scientific background of the medical doctor, but this increase in science has been achieved at the expense of the art that is clinical medicine.

The sophistication of medical education has been copied by the chiropractic profession. So, too, have the inherent drawbacks. Overall, this trend has had a positive effect on chiropractic, but the drawbacks need to be eliminated by both professions.

The greatest benefit the allopathic profession has bestowed on chiropractic is adversity. Although it has slowed our growth, it has caused chiropractors to concentrate their skills in treating their patients and measuring up to the challenge of survival. The staying power of the chiropractic profession is found in its principles and philosophy. It is these very principles that will correct the deficiencies of chiropractic education and insure the continued growth of chiropractic.

Before discussing the principles of chiropractic philosophy, it should be pointed out that philosophy is a metaphysical concept. It serves as a purpose and reinforcement for clinical practice. The basis of clinical practice is a thorough knowledge of anatomy, physiology and biomechanics.

The principles that follow are listed out of respect for our chiropractic heritage. When our knowledge of the subjects related to the human body was limited, it was these principles that enabled chiropractors to treat the sick. Discussion of all these principles can be found in the works of Ralph Stephenson, D.C. and F.P. DeGiacomo, D.C. The discussion in this book will center around six principles. These are the principles that can directly be applied to the treatment of any patient.

1. THE MAJOR PREMISE
   A universal intelligence is in all matter and continually gives to it all its properties and actions, thus maintaining it in existence.
2. THE CHIROPRACTIC MEANING OF LIFE
   The expression of this intelligence through matter is the chiropractic meaning of life.
3. THE UNION OF INTELLIGENCE AND MATTER
   Life is necessarily the union of intelligence and matter.
4. THE TRIUNE OF LIFE
   Life is a truinity having three necessary united factors, namely Intelligence, Force and Matter.
5. THE PERFECTION OF THE TRUINE
   In order to have 100% life, there must be 100% intelligence, 100% force and 100% matter.
6. THE PRINCIPLE OF TIME
   There is no process that does not require time.
7. THE AMOUNT OF INTELLIGENCE IN MATTER
   The amount of intelligence for any given amount of matter is 100%, and is always proportional to its requirements.
8. THE FUNCTION OF INTELLIGENCE
   The function of intelligence is to create force.
9. THE AMOUNT OF FORCE CREATED BY INTELLIGENCE
   The amount of force is to unite intelligence and matter.

10. THE FUNCTION OF FORCE

The function of force is to unite intelligence and matter.

11. THE CHARACTER OF UNIVERSAL FORCES

The forces of universal intelligence are manifested by physical laws; are unserving and unadapted, and have no solicitude for the structures in which they work.

12. INTERFERENCE WITH TRANSMISSION OF UNIVERSAL FORCES

There can be interference with transmission of universal forces.

13. THE FUNCTION OF MATTER

The function of matter is to express force.

14. UNIVERSAL LIFE

Force is manifested by motion in matter; all matter has motion, therefore there is universal life in all matter.

15. NO MOTION WITHOUT THE EFFORT OF FORCE

Matter can have no motion without the application of force by intelligence.

16. INTELLIGENCE IN BOTH ORGANIC AND INORGANIC MATTER

Universal intelligence gives force to both organic and inorganic matter.

17. CAUSE AND EFFECT

Every effect has a cause and every cause has effects.

18. EVIDENCE OF LIFE

The signs of life are evidence of the intelligence of life.

19. ORGANIC MATTER

The material of the body of a "living thing" is organized matter.

20. INNATE INTELLIGENCE

A "living thing" has as inborn intelligence within its body, called Innate Intelligence.

21. THE MISSION OF INNATE INTELLIGENCE

The mission of Innate Intelligence is to maintain the material of the body of the "living thing" in active organization.

22. THE AMOUNT OF INNATE INTELLIGENCE

There is 100% of Innate Intelligence in every "living thing" the requisite amount, proportional to its organization.

23. THE FUNCTION OF INNATE INTELLIGENCE

The function of Innate Intelligence is to adapt universal forces and matter for use in the body, so that all parts of the body will have co-ordinated action for mutual benefit.

24. THE LIMITS OF ADAPTATION
Innate Intelligence adapts forces and matter for the body as long as it can do so without breaking a universal law, or Innate Intelligence is limited by the limitation of matter.

25. THE CHARACTER OF INNATE FORCES
The forces of Innate Intelligence never injure or destory the structures in which they work.

26. COMPARISON OF UNIVERSAL OR INNATE FORCES
In order to carry on the universal cycle of life, Universal forces are destructive and Innate forces constructive, as regards structural matter.

27. THE NORMALITY OF INNATE INTELLIGENCE
Innate Intelligence is always normal and its function is always normal.

28. THE CONDUCTORS OF INNATE FORCES
The forces of Innate Intelligence operate through or over the nervous system in animal bodies.

29. There can be interference with the transmission of Innate forces.

30. THE CAUSE OF DISEASE
Interference with the transmission of Innate forces causes incoordination of disease.

31. SUBLUXATIONS
Interference with transmission in the body is always directly or indirectly due to subluxations in the spinal column.

32. THE PRINCIPLE OF COORDINATION
Coordination is the principle of harmonious action of all the parts of an organism, in fulfilling their offices and purposes.

33. THE LAW OF DEMAND AND SUPPLY
The law of demand and supply is existent in the body in its ideal state; wherein the "clearing house" is the brain, Innate the virtuous "banker", brain cells "clerks", and nerve cells "messengers".

1. A UNIVERSAL INTELLIGENCE IS IN ALL MATTER, AND CONTINUALLY GIVES TO IT ALL ITS PROPERTIES AND ACTIONS, THUS MAINTAINING IT IN EXISTENCE.

In healing there has always been an acknowledgement that there is a force or power that supersedes the doctor and the patient. In ancient times, physicians invoked the gods to intervene on behalf of their patients and restore health. Nowadays, this faith has been directed towards science. Religion, like philosophy, is removed from science. As the world became more scientific and specialized, subjects which seemed incompatible with the progressive nature of science were relegated to an insignificant role in a person's education. Science produced results and phenomena that people could see, hear and touch; religion and philosophy could make no such claim; therefore, they were lost to a position of secondary importance.

Science taught society how to achieve results for immediate gratification, but did little to answer questions regarding the purpose of life. If there is a purpose to life, what is it? Science has its part in the scheme of life, and although it can give mechanical and technical answers as to why an event has occurred, it is not the only source of an answer to this complex question.

Because so much emphasis has been placed on the power of science and the skill and education of doctors, both doctors and patients have lost their perspective regarding health. The prevalent attitude is that the doctor has the power to cure and the patient has no power at all. In reality, a doctor-patient relationship is as symbiotic as any natural relationship that has both partners benefiting from the arrangement. A patient gives the doctor the opportunity to practice skills taught in school. A doctor affords the patient a chance to regain health. Each day the master of the universe unfolds, and each day doctors and patients assume their roles in this occurrence.

The intelligence that maintains order in the universe is the source of healing. There is no disgrace in a doctor acknowledging a power superior to his own. This acknowledgement of a force or power pervading the universe should serve as a reminder that the skill of a physician facilitates healing, it does not create the process. It should also be remembered that because the source of healing is universal in nature, it is not the property of any one branch of the healing arts, and a cure can best be effected by practicing within the natural confines of our ability.

There is no way of knowing how many worlds exist in the universe. We can only be responsible for this world. Each patient, although a unique individual, is part of a bigger picture of life. The well-being of an individual can be seen as an increase in productivity of neighborhoods, communities, cities, states, countries and the world. To render competent care to a patient is to improve the quality of life in society, thereby improving the nature of our environment.

2. THE FORCES OF UNIVERSAL INTELLIGENCE ARE MANIFESTED BY PHYSICAL LAWS, ARE UNSWERVING

AND UNADAPTED, AND HAVE NOT SOLICITUDE FOR THE STRUCTURE IN WHICH THEY WORK.

This principle reinforces the concept that man is subservient to the powers of the universe. To a degree these forces can be controlled, but only insofar as this control does not prohibit the mainfestation of the universal plan. This plan continually unfolds, at its own pace, without the intervention of man. This being the case, man is not as important as he believes himself to be, but instead, is another creature, another aspect of life that moves in time. This progression of time continually occurs on all levels of life, from the single celled amoeba, to the cerebrum of man. From the most active of organisms to the most stationary of objects, life unfolds. Although each new adventure seems important within the context of the world in which it occurs, it is minor with regard to the universal plan.

To accept a role as a viable part of life lends a new and different perspective to daily routine. There are certain laws which have been proposed by science that are applicable to philosophy. The first law states, energy is neither created nor destroyed, but changes form. Each person, at one time or another, is said to be in his own little world. That is because each person's existence is a little world. At the beginning of time there was X amount of energy dispersed throughout all the organisms and objects in existence. According to scientific law, that same amount of energy still exists, although it may not be in the same form that it was first manifested. With this in mind, consider that each human being is energy and maintains a place in the universal plan. Consider that the goal of each human being is to learn and experience as much as possible before undergoing the period of transition known as death, Although death marks the end of life as we perceive it, according to science, it is nothing more than a state that will enable that which was at one time a human life, to change into another form. This transition being what it is, life does not end with death; it simply changes.

There are always some unfortunate tragedies taking place somewhere on this planet. The situation seems unjust and cruel and without purpose. Perhaps the purpose of these challenges is that they are the necessary experiences that afford the individual involved the opportunity to learn something about himself, and then move on to new adventures.

A second law of science states that for every action, there is an equal and opposite reaction. Thus the laws of science confirm the philosophical concept of harmony in nature. No life is made up of only pain, nor is a life exclusively made up of happiness.

There is a necessity for being able to experience a variety of emotions, because there will naturally occur a balance in their dispersement.

The function of a chiropractor is to remember this concept of balance. A patient usually presents with some degree of pain. To treat patients on a daily basis and focus only on their pain is a frustrating and emotionally draining experience. Likewise, to tell a patient to learn to enjoy from their pain is not conducive to building a practice that will treat many people. But to treat patients with sensitivity and empathy, and not lose sight of the fact that these painful situations are finite in nature, takes the pressure of making an instantaneous correction away from the chiropractor, and allows him to fully practice the art of healing.

Also, to tell a patient his pain is part of the universal plan might not comfort him. Although that might well be the case, it is not in the best interest of the patient to tell him this when he is in pain. A chiropractor has no more insight into the universal plan than any other person. Chiropractors might be more sensitive to it, but they do not possess an in-depth knowledge of it. Chiropractors can best help the universal plan by applying the science, art and philosophy to their patients. In this way, they will facilitate healing in their patients. If through corrected health the quality of life a person is experiencing improves, he can better function in the attainment of his personal goals. Those universal plans that need be achieved will be, whether or not a person is cognizant of his role.

3. A LIVING THING HAS AN INBORN INTELLIGENCE WITHIN ITS BODY CALLED INNATE INTELLIGENCE.

That part of an individual that we most relate to, both personally and professionally, is the patient's innate intelligence. It is this inborn intelligence that utilizes an adjustment to balance homeostatic mechanisms and allow the patient to fulfill his destiny.

There is a normal balance within an individual, a balance that has been functional since conception. It has determined the sequence that the new life developed, giving attention, when appropriate, to the nervous system, heart, blood vessels, bones and muscle. It has been able to adjust itself to the needs of the individual without the benefit of outside intervention. It is a function of the chiropractor, when homeostasis is thrown into a state of imbalance, to utilize his skill and knowledge to reinstate the balance so it can properly function and administer to the needs of the individual. Why is it that innate intelligence functioned so accurately in the womb, and once in society, must be aided by doctors? The answer is simple. In a natural setting life progresses in a natural sequence, uninhibited by any devices of man. Society is far from a natural setting. Instead it breeds situations which can easily overcome an individual's normal physiological resistance and necessitate some form of external intervention.

Universal intelligence maintains order in the universe, and innate intelligence maintains order within an individual. Unfortunately, society is maintained by educated intelligence. This educated intelligence has helped pervert natural instincts regarding health and has distorted the basic values which are conducive to peaceful living. This situation has taken many years to evolve, and there is no direct answer to the dilemma. The only significant contribution that can be made in changing these attitudes is effectively treating individuals so they can, in turn, make positive contributions towards society.

There is no chance that society will ever improve itself to a point where there is no need for doctors. But a situation can be realized where the role of a doctor is seen as being adjunctive to a patient's health as opposed to the source of a patient's health.

4. INNATE INTELLIGENCE IS LIMITED BY THE LIMITATION OF MATTER.

Unlike universal intelligence, whose power is dispersed throughout the cosmos, innate intelligence is concentrated within individuals. Innate intelligence is linked with universal intelligence, but is subordinate to it, and does not possess the same resources. Not possessing the same resources, and being under the influence of universal laws lends to each life an aura of mortality.

It is the purpose of innate intelligence to maintain a functioning life. When the body malfunctions, the inherent recuperative powers of the body are stimulated and affect the natural healing process that enables the body to contain and eliminate the disease state. These recuperative powers are manifested through tissue which is finite in ability and nature. Each time a patient is treated there is no guarantee that a response in the form of healing will take place.

There is a finite quality to everything that concerns being human. This does not exclude a doctor's knowledge and ability and includes a patient's ability to heal. When one considers how many times a human heart beats in a lifetime, or how fast a neural impulse travels, or how many cells make up the brain, there is a sense of awe and respect for the power and majesty of life. No machine on earth possesses the qualities of the human body, and no machine on earth is as cognizant of its mortality.

Each person lives an undetermined amount of time. Each person will change during this period of time. Chiropractors can only hope to help their patients stay functional and productive throughout life.

5. THERE IS NO PROCESS THAT DOES NOT REQUIRE TIME.

In a world inundated with fast food franchises, split second computers and technology that will span countries and continents in a matter of minutes, it is hard for doctors and patients to accept that all things, especially the healing process, take time. In a society that is dominated by material and financial compensation, it is no wonder we have no patience for the necessity of time in the natural healing process of the body. In general, people would rather sacrifice their health than their money or possessions.

When the body is not functioning at the maximum, it should not be expected to, nor can it, achieve its normal productivity. Whether or not there is a conscious acknowledgement of a patient's ill health on the part of the doctor or the patient, the body's inability to perform will reinforce the fact that the patient is ill.

Patients must be educated that their health did not change in a matter of minutes, but, instead, has continually and progressively developed into a state that has necessitated external intervention. The human body was not created to endure and tolerate pain, although it can if the need arises. Pain is meant to be a signal that there is a malfunction within the body. It now becomes the goal of the doctor-patient relationship to correct the imbalance and restore health.

The patient who presents to an office after a trauma has a direct cause-effect relationship to his problem. Granted the time factor that is required to enable the patient to feel better is unknown, because when the patient understands the cause of the problem he is more tolerant of the healing process and its required time. Unfortunately, such a direct cause-effect relationship cannot be made with the ill-postured patient who comes in with a chronic low back condition. The patient's body is a reflection of a life that has been less than the person's dreams and expectations. Now, through the skill of the chiropractor, and the cooperation of the patient, a healing process must be initiated that will alleviate the musculoskeletal conditions present, and enable the patient to face the challenges of life from a position of health, as opposed to disease.

There are factors that influence the amount of time required in the healing process. Among them are the skill of the chiropractor, the attitude and cooperation of the patient, and the stresses placed upon the patient. Because a chiropractor can only be responsible for the doctor's skill, it is unfair to project a specific amount of time to alleviate a patient's condition. It is equally unfair for a patient to expect that a doctor's skill is the only determinant in their condition.

Time is a universal concept that has been given parameters by man. To this end, man finds himself controlled by time. There is no such thing as a second, minute, hour, day, week, month, or year. These are man made parameters, devised to control or at least give some order to daily living. In this effort to control time, man has become controlled. Many people are distressed because they mark birthdays not as significant days to commemorate accomplishments, but as a period of meditation to ponder those things they have not achieved.

6. COORDINATION IS THE PRINCIPLE OF HARMONIOUS ACTION OF ALL PARTS OF THE ORGANISM IN FULFILLING THEIR PURPOSE.

This is the principle of holistic healing, the principle that links chiropractic with Hippocrates. It was Hippocrates who stressed that man should be studied in his entirety and in relation to his environment. He also proposed that homeostasis is reached only when man lives in harmony with his external environment.

The human body is an integrated organism. There is no one part of the body that does not affect the functioning of the other parts. Chiropractors must keep in mind that they are treating a whole human being, not just the spine and musculoskeletal system. People are complex, yet simple. Situations affect different people in different ways, but the end result is that everyone wants to be happy and comfortable. Though there are conditions that are painful and unhappy, they can best be tolerated within a healthy body.

It is a function of a chiropractor, utilizing his knowledge and skill, to help patients maintain the harmonious action that is an innate characteristic of life. As long as this harmonious action is maintained, the organism can fulfill its purpose in life.

By acknowledging the need of coordination in maintaining the welfare of the organism, there is indicated the need for astute observation and diagnosis on the part of the chiropractor. It is the function of the chiropractor to facilitate healing in a patient entrusted to his care; it is his obligation to treat the patient, if he has determined this to be the patient's need, or refer the patient to the appropriate member of the healing arts.

EPILOGUE

The effective application of chiropractic principles in clinical practice is the unique characteristic that separates the chiropractor from the allopath. It is this blending of science and philosophy that allows the chiropractor to approach patients with a human quality that has never been consistently duplicated by any other profession. The chiropractic approach is undiluted with the pretense of scientific jargon that separates the patient, a person, from the doctor, another person. A chiropractor who is enthusiastic about his work shares this enthusiasm with his patients. In turn, patients share their lives with their chiropractor, and the result is doctor-patient relationship that is alive.

> "Clinical medicine should be regarded neither as an art nor a science by itself, but as a special kind of relationship between two people, a doctor and a patient..."
>
> Ashely Montagu

Those decisions that a chiropractor make which affect a patient's life should be made on two levels. First, ample consideration should be given to the personal, occupational and social conditions under which the patient lives. Secondly, the chiropractor must rely on his clinical expertise to accurately diagnose the patient's problem and plot the proper course of treatment.

> "The real work of a doctor is only faintly realized by many lay people. It is not an affair of health centres or public clinics or operating theatres, or laboratories or hospital beds. These techniques have their place in medicine, but they are not medicine. The essential unit of medical practice is the occasion when, in the privacy and intimacy of the consulting room or the sick room, a person who is ill, or who believes himself to be ill, seeks the advice of a doctor whom he trusts. This is a consultation and all else in medicine derives from it."
>
> Sir James Spence

Three items should be kept in mind in directing the advancement of chiropractic:

1. Allopaths should no longer be allowed to dictate the rules. The chiropractic profession and the allopathic profession are two distinct entities. Therefore, the abilities of each profession should be

assessed differently. These professions should be respected for their unique qualities.

There will be times when it is necessary to call upon the services of an allopath or surgeon. If the clinical indications are such that a referral of this nature is in the best interest of the patient, it should be made without hesitation. Perhaps it is time that the allopathic profession learns from our example.

2. Individual chiropractic efforts should be made towards producing unparallelled clinical results. The real work of a chiropractor is getting sick people well. This can only be achieved through the proper application of the science, art, and philosophy of chiropractic.

The detached "professional" approach of treating patients does not lend itself to uncovering all the facts that influence a patient's health. It would be in the best interest of chiropractic if chiropractors remembered the original meanings of the words doctor and physician. Those original definitions are still functional in the clinical sense.

3. Analyze which direction our educational system is going and direct it towards those objectives which are in the best interest of the public and the profession. If it is determined that the educational process is emphasizing one aspect of the chiropractic triune, perhaps it is time to institute balance to the system.

As society has become enamoured with science, so too has chiropractic education. Based on the results of science to date, and the quality of life that has accompanied these results, I question whether such emphasis should be placed on one aspect of chiropractic. Putting too much emphasis there throws the entire foundation of the profession into a state of imbalance, which we know is incompatible with health, and in this case growth.

There is a need for science. Any doctor who does not possess a functional knowledge of science and purports to be a chiropractor is a fraud. Likewise, any chiropractor who does not have a functional knowledge of the principles and philosophy of chiropractic is equally fraudulent. The triune of science, art and philosophy must be kept in balance if chiropractic is to grow and affect the health of society and fulfill its destiny.

After struggling through years of regimented education; after having been brainwashed by media propaganda espousing the superhuman nature and infallibility of doctors; and after being constantly reminded by society that there is an image that must be maintained, it is no wonder doctors lose sight of the essence of clinical practice. Education and its infatuation with science has deprived the doctor of his most powerful ally, his humanity. The ability to possess knowledge and skill, yet maintain faith in the intuitive ability of human instincts, is rare. All too often a patient lauds a physician's skill, but finds him lacking as a person. A doctor cannot be lacking either in his technical skill and knowledge, nor in his humanism, because the combination of the two is what makes a doctor. Technical skill alone makes a person a technician. Despite any title he might possess, the shortsighted, limited scope with which a patient is viewed can only be the observation of a technician. Combining this technical skill with sensitivity and empathy transforms the technician into a doctor.

Part of chiropractic art is being a doctor. This art can only be realized when a physician has enough confidence and skill so as not to be threatened by a patient's questions or to be unsympathetic to a patient's needs. More than anything else, a doctor needs to be human in his approach to patients.

The ideas contained on the previous pages are by no means an exhaustive study on the topics covered. They are a somewhat superficial compilation of many of the facts that have influenced the American approach to health. More than that, they have been compiled as a reminder to our innate sense of honesty that our direction with regard to health has been in error.

Chiropractors have their work cut out for them. They must be able to re-educate a public that is already programmed in health habits. This is not an easy task, but is one that can be accomplished.

Before attempting to change public attitudes, chiropractors must undergo some self reflection. The deficiencies of the allopathic approach have been outlined. Which ones have been copied by chiropractors? This is a question only individual chiropractors can answer. It is easy to fall into the trap of following in the path of a profession that has produced results, even though the quality of those results is in question. In our effort to survive we have allowed the allopath to dictate the rules. Prove what you do scientifically. Come up to our standards.

Imitation is the highest form of flattery. By imitating and emulating allopathic procedures, we lend credibility to their claim as being the legitimate leaders of the healing arts. If the results produced by allopaths were truly extraordinary, there would be no reason not to follow their example. This is not the case. The allopathic approach was formulated with the best interests of the public at heart. But because the reason for the development of an attitude is of noble nature, it does not mean the movement itself is without flaw. The pied piper allopath has played his song and the chiropractors have followed. There is no disgrace in being human and making a mistake. In terms of health, society moved in a direction.

As with any movement, in the beginning, there are high ideals and aspirations. Only once in progress can an evaluation be made. To make a mistake is acceptable. To realize that there are shortcomings to an approach and try to make the approach valid by continuing its use is unforgivable.

Now is the time to honestly assess our position. Those efforts made to help the growth of chiropractic should continue. Those mistakes made should be corrected.

There are those who might feel that my treatment of the allopathic profession is somewhat harsh. The facts contained herein were not written as an indictment of clinical allopathy, for which I have high regard, but rather as an exposition of some of the lesser known facts that have helped determine our present health attitudes.

Finally, I hope the ideas contained in this book have caused the reader to reflect on his contributions to the situations mentioned. There are as many interpretations of philosophy as there are human beings. If my thoughts have in any way made sense to you, or have reinforced some of your beliefs, fine. If you consider my thoughts irrelevant, or they make you angry, that was not my intention. My only request is that you think about your feelings honestly and consider how you have gotten to a point in life where you can stop listening or learning from the opinion of others. The principles referred to throughout this book have been discussed from the viewpoint of their clinical relevance. If the discussion was not of a limited scope, we would notice that the principles of chiropractic are not only the backbone of the chiropractic profession, they are a unique way of approaching life.

REFERENCES

American Chiropractic Associates - Chiropractic State of Arts Department of Public Affairs - 1977

F.P. DeGiacomo - Man's Greatest Gift to Man - L.S.R. Learning Associates Inc., Old Bethpage, New York, N.Y. 11804 - 1978

Rene Dubos - Mirage of Health - Harper & Row, Publishers, Inc.- 1971

Jack Lapatra - Healing - McGraw-Hill Book Co. - 1978

Michael J. Lepore, M.D. - Death of the Clinician Requiem or Reveille? - Publisher Charles C. Thomas - 1982

Richard M. Magraw, M.D. - Daniel B. Magraw, M.B.A. - Ferment in Medicine - Published by W.B. Saunders Company - 1966

Robert S. Mendelsohn, M.D. - Confessions of a Medical Heretic - Published by Contemporary Books, Inc. - 1979

R.W. Stephenson - Chiropractic Text Book - Published by The Palmer School of Chiropractic - 1948

"ILL HEALTH, OF BODY OR OF MIND, IS DEFEAT . . . HEALTH ALONE IS VICTORY. LET ALL MEN, IF THEY CAN MANAGE IT, CONTRIVE TO BE HEALTHY."

—THOMAS CARLYLE